Exploring Egbert

Learning by experience

Created by Luke Thompson

Co-author Caroline Bennett

Illustrated by Kat Willott

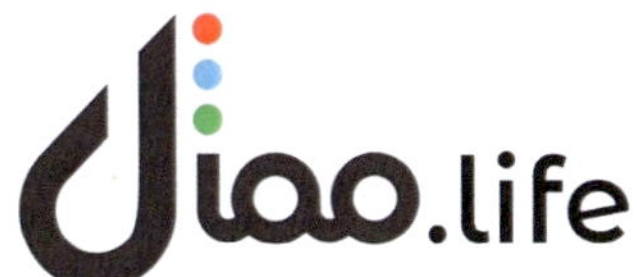

Published by Jiao Ltd

Jiao.life

Scan the QR codes to access the digital book or listen to the audio book.

Audiobook

Digital Book

The Seven Stages of Switch Development

Exploring Egbert is part of the Switch Heroes, social stories created to support switch-users with their Switch progression. The Switch Heroes series is part of the Seven Stages of Switch Development, created by Occupational Therapist and AT specialist Luke Thompson.

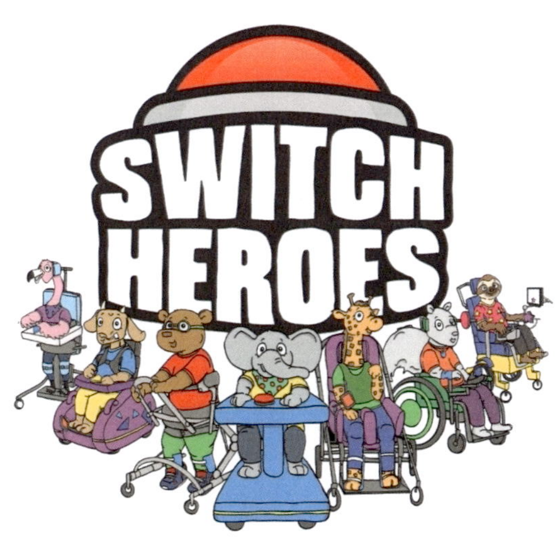

It's Egbert the Explorer!

Has he come to play?

I wonder what things

He will do today?

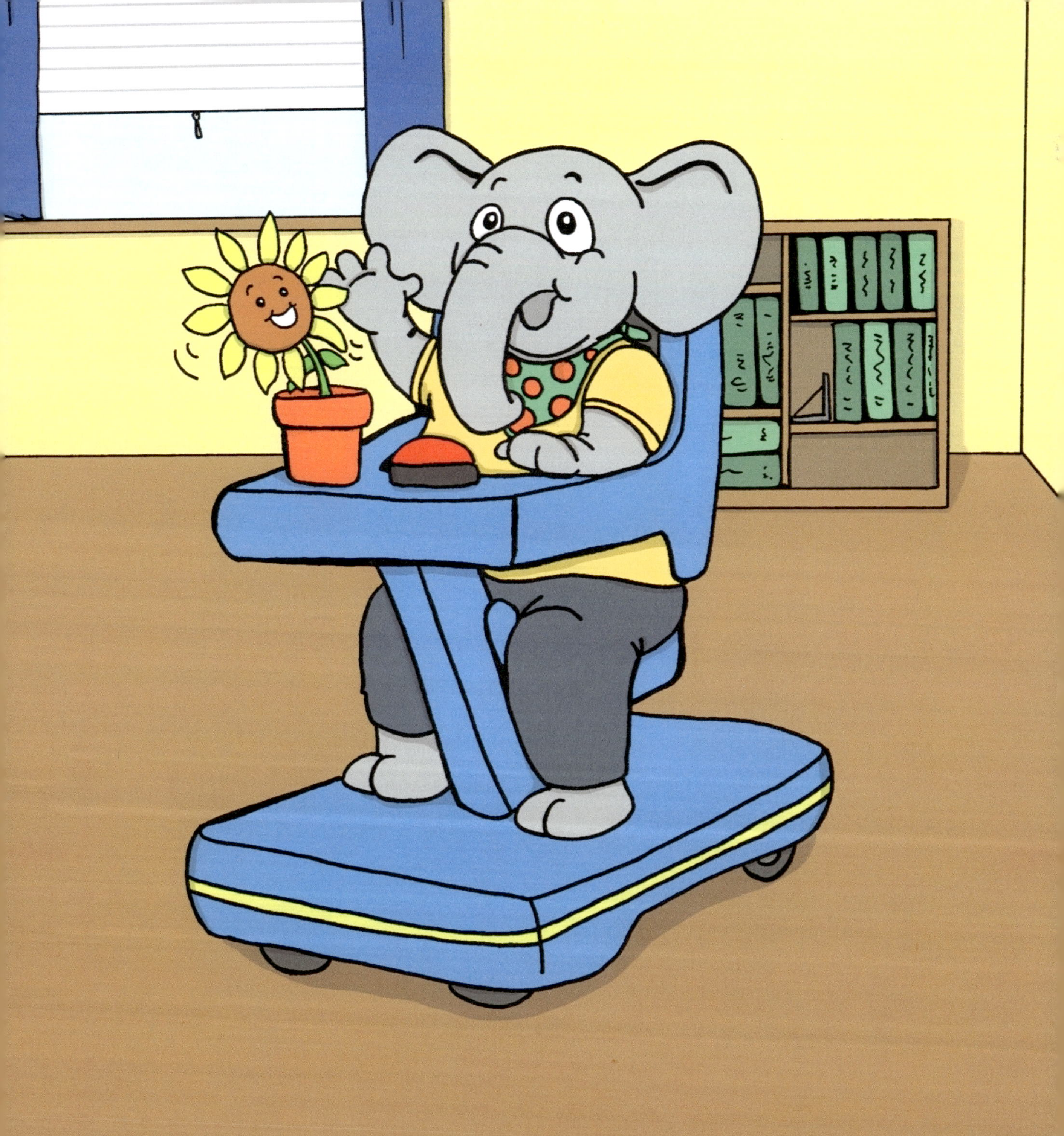

He has something special
Sitting on his chair
It's red and round
and looks exciting!
"What's that Egbert?
Why's it there?"

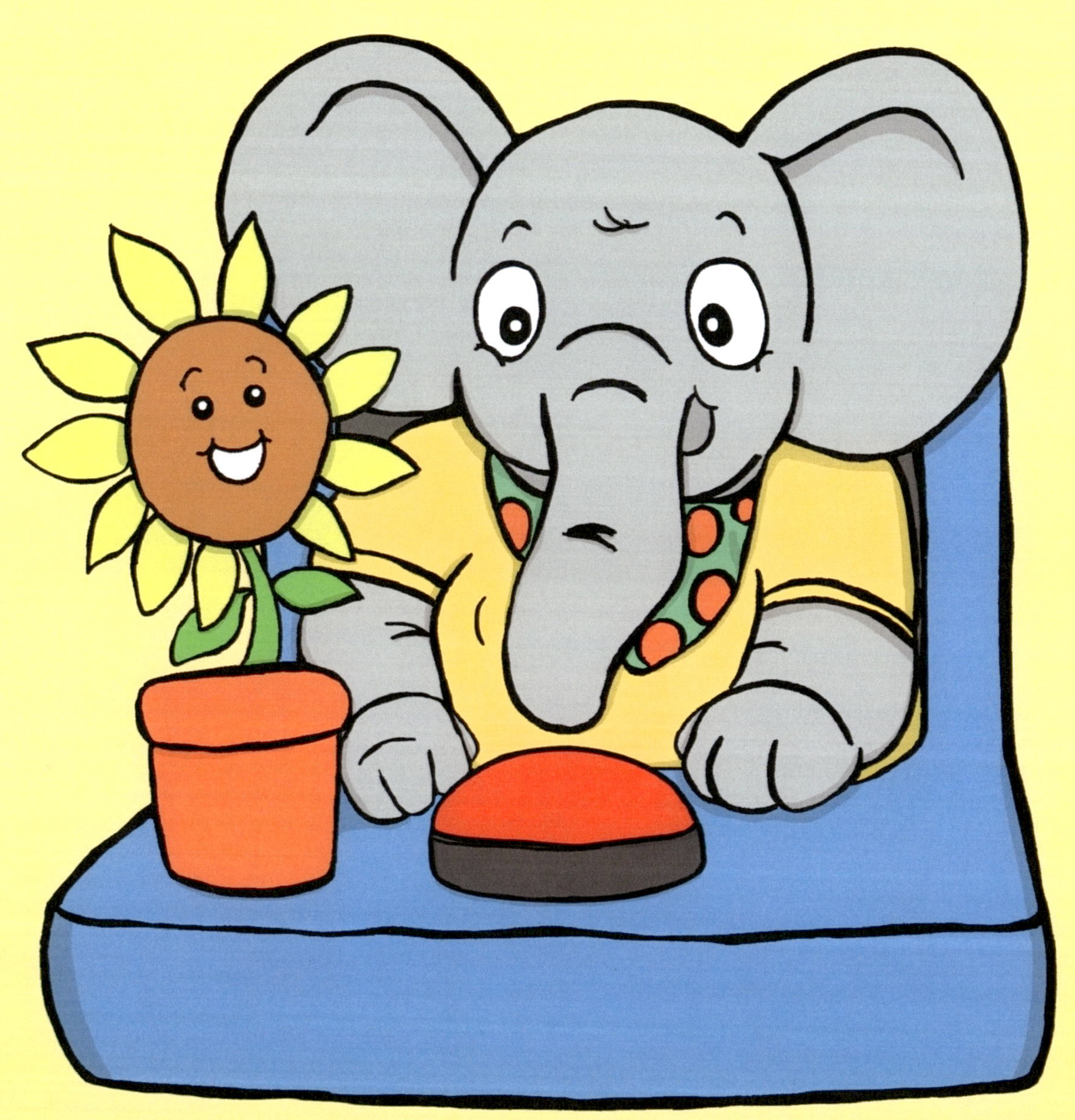

Egbert shows off his button
"It's a switch my friend
And when I push it down
The toy will start to bend"

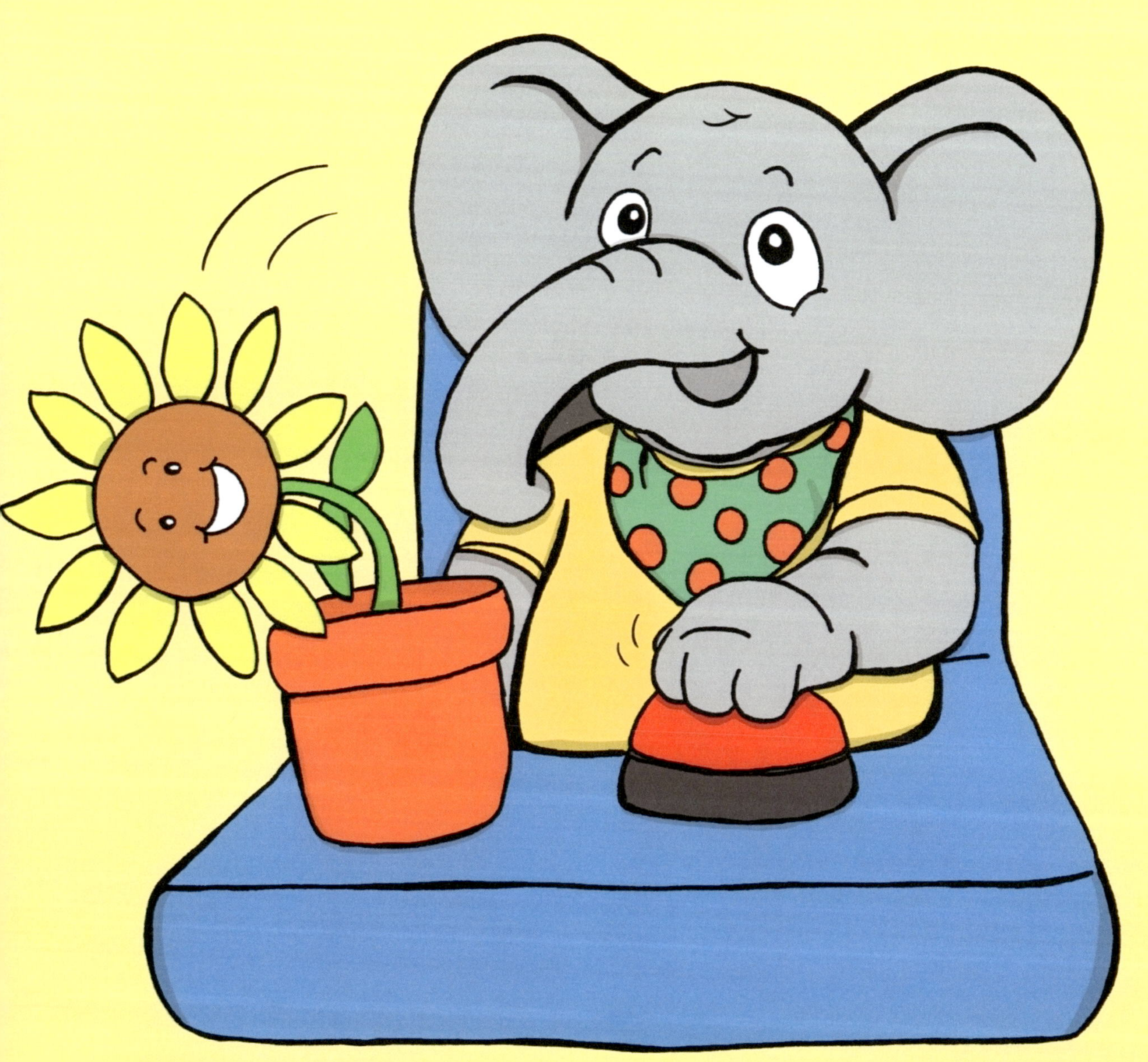

"The Switch is very clever
I use it how I can
Push it with your head, your foot
Even with your hand"

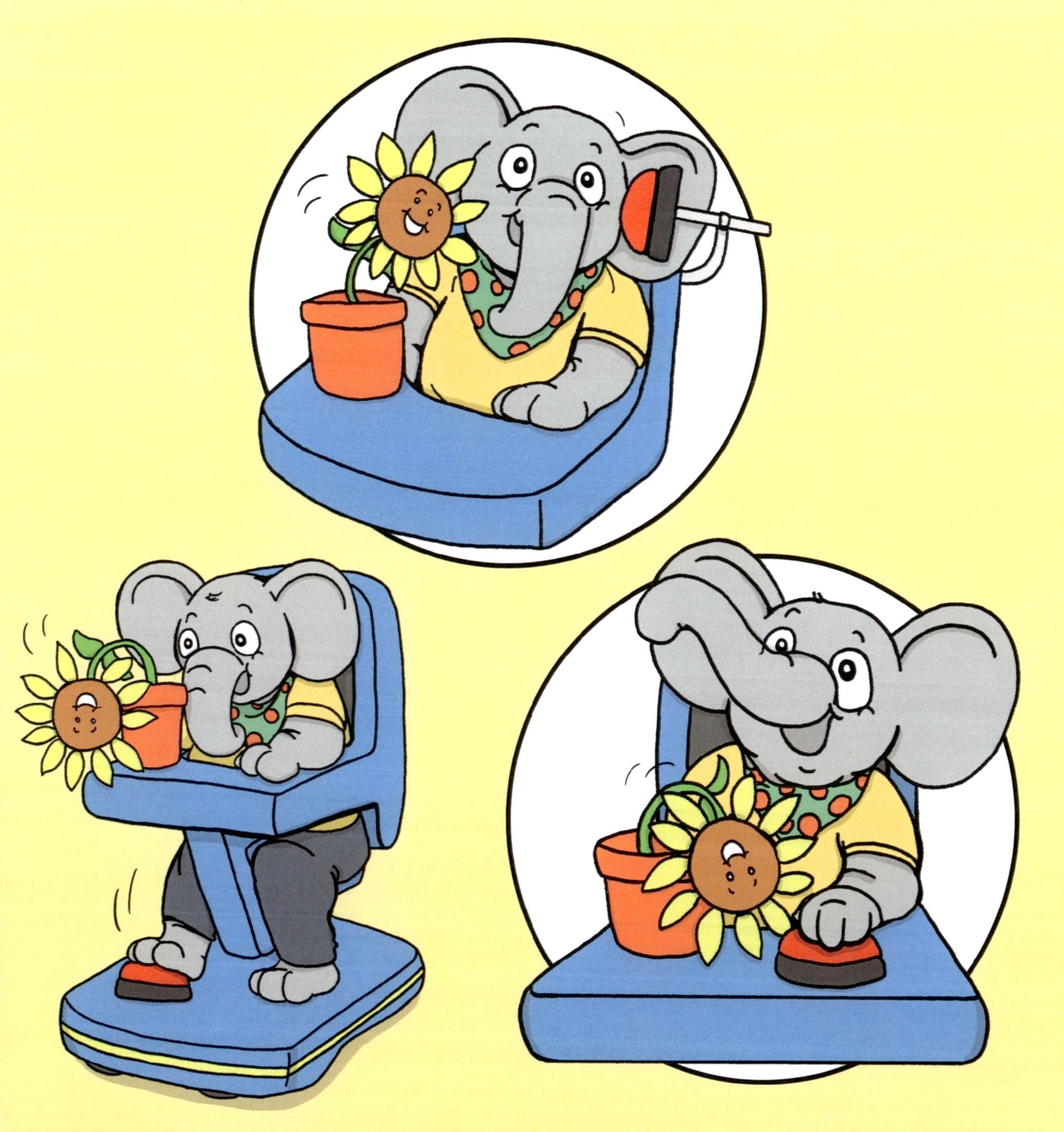

"When you use this switch
It starts to play a song
And change the colour of the light
Try it! You can't go wrong"

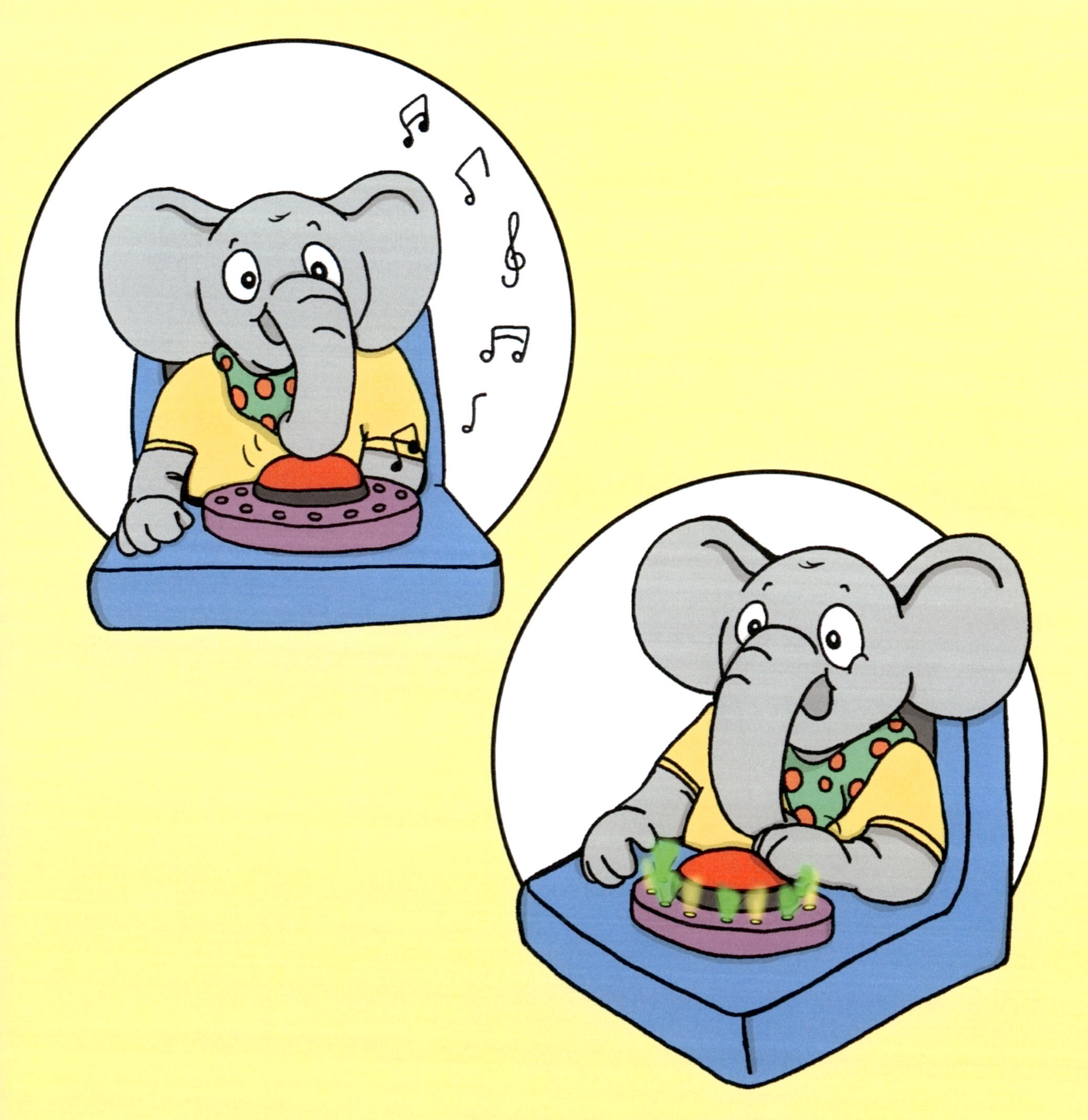

"It takes a little practice
Have a go! Have fun!
Once you've learnt to do it
Your switch journey's begun"

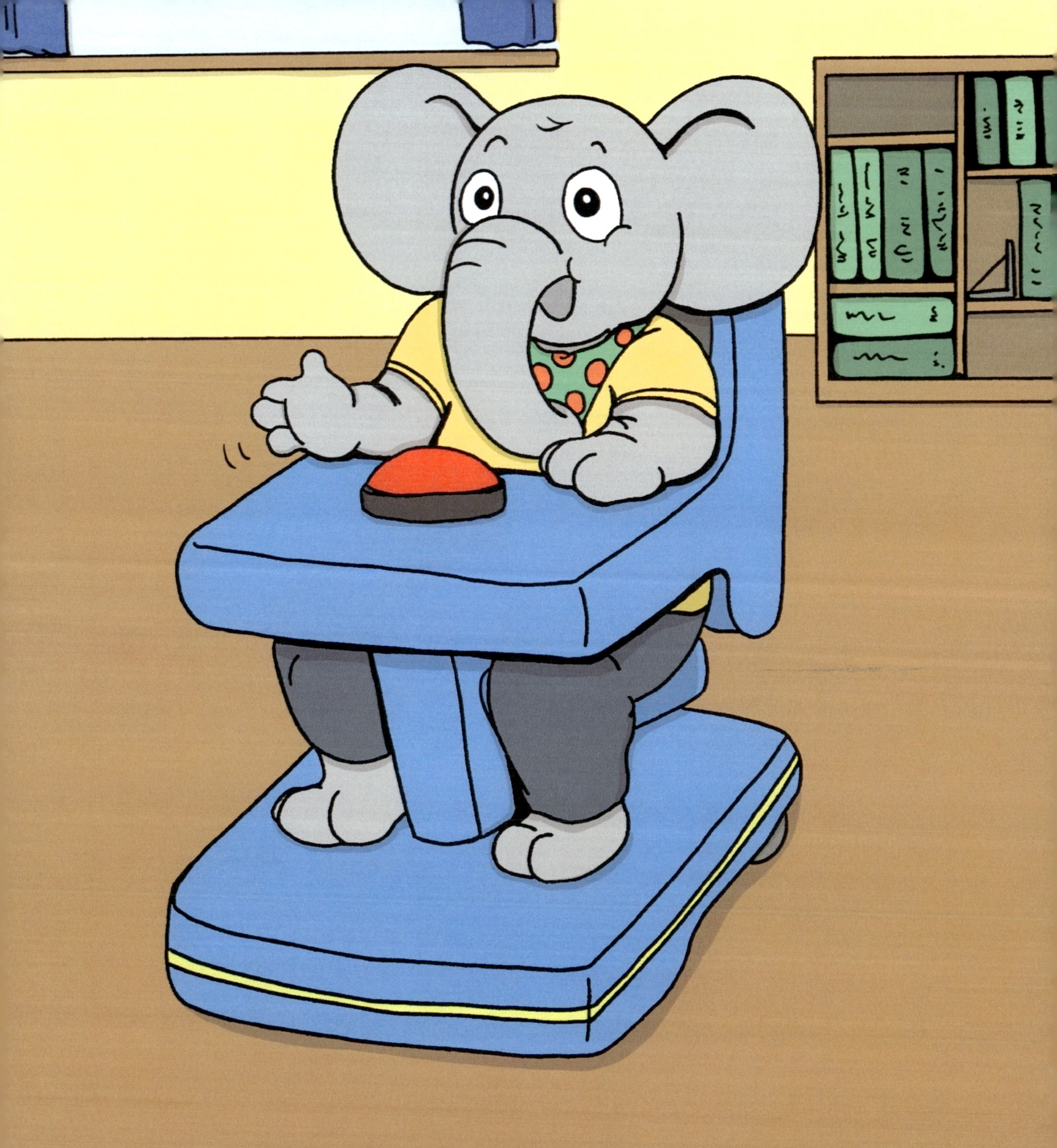

Oh, thank you, Egbert

We've started to explore

And try our big red button

We're much braver than before!

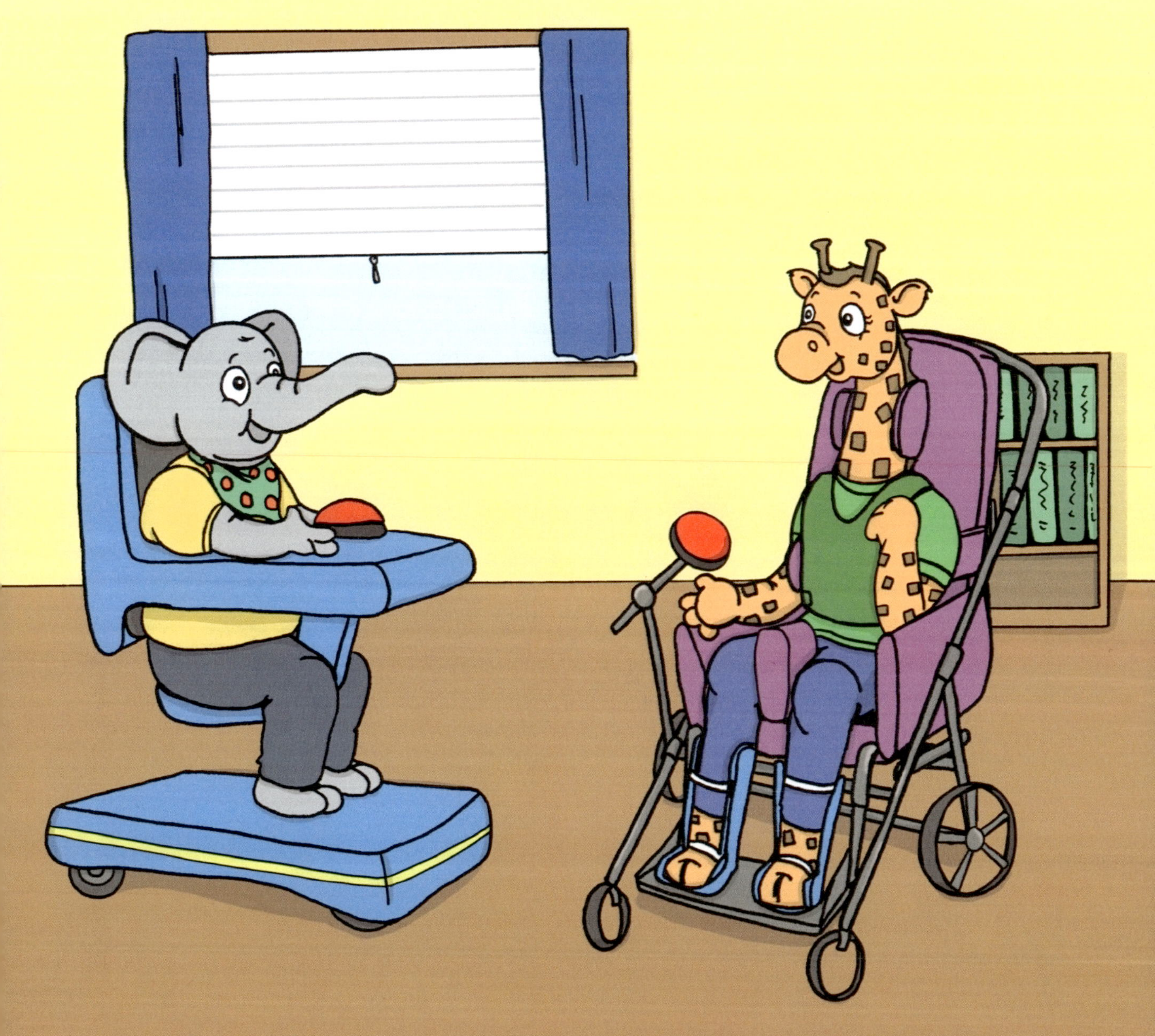

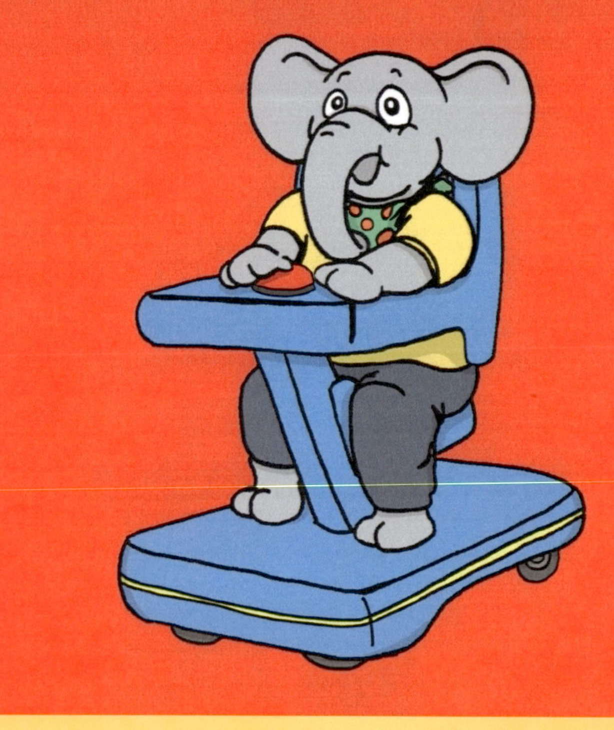
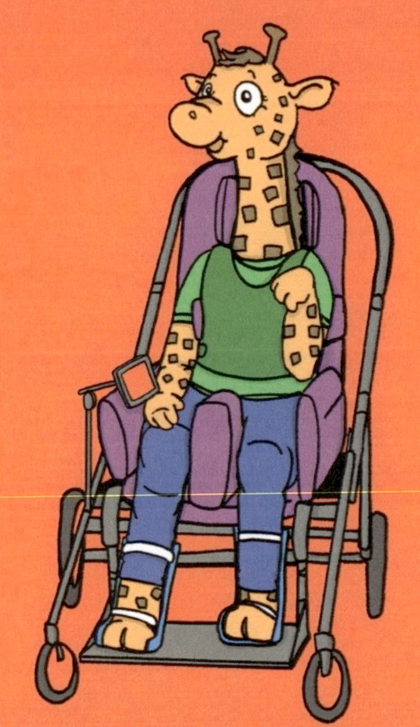
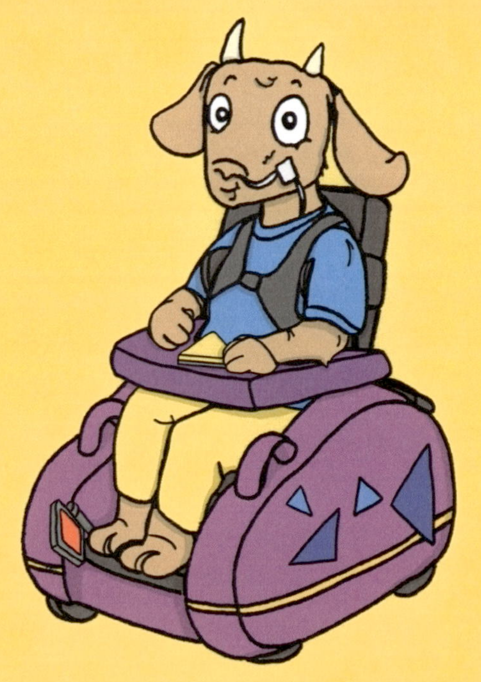
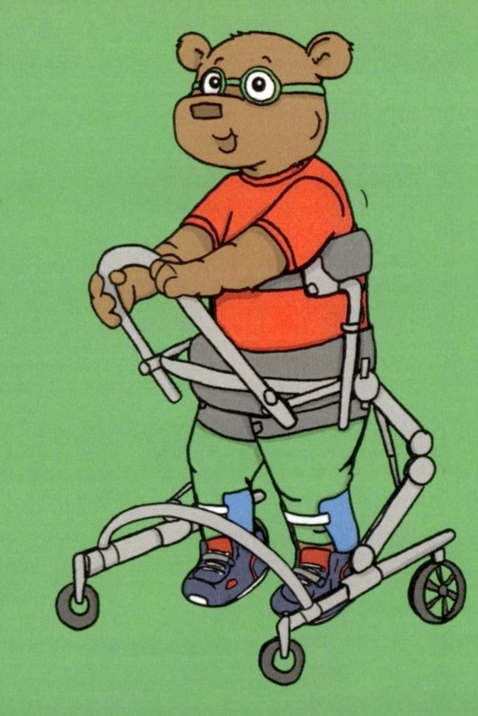

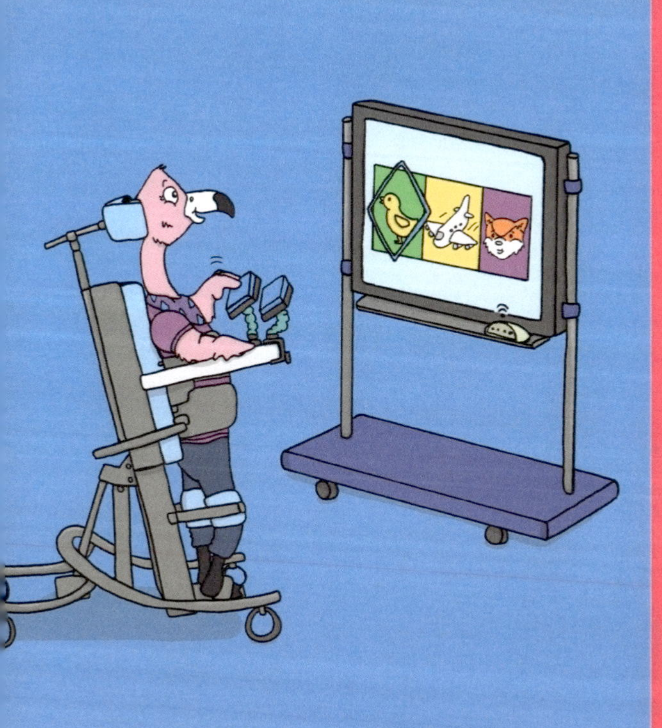

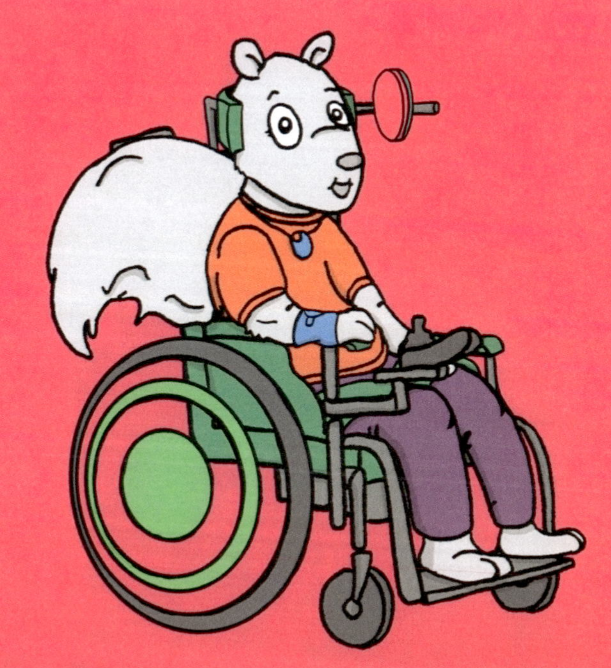

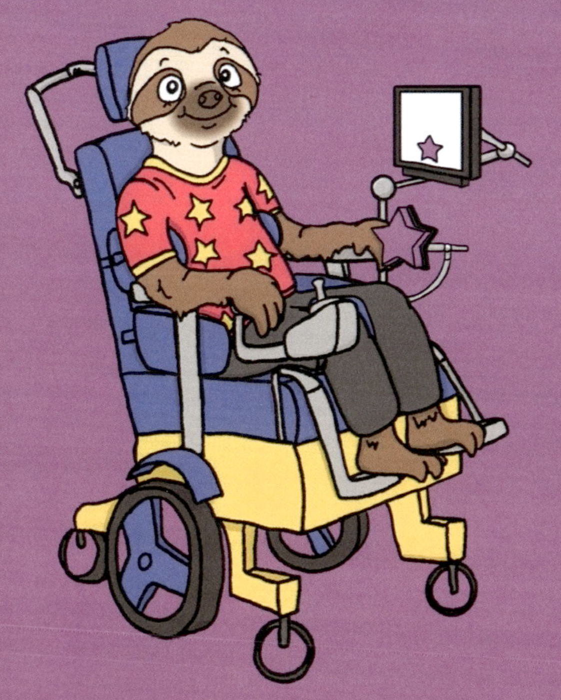

Photo of you!

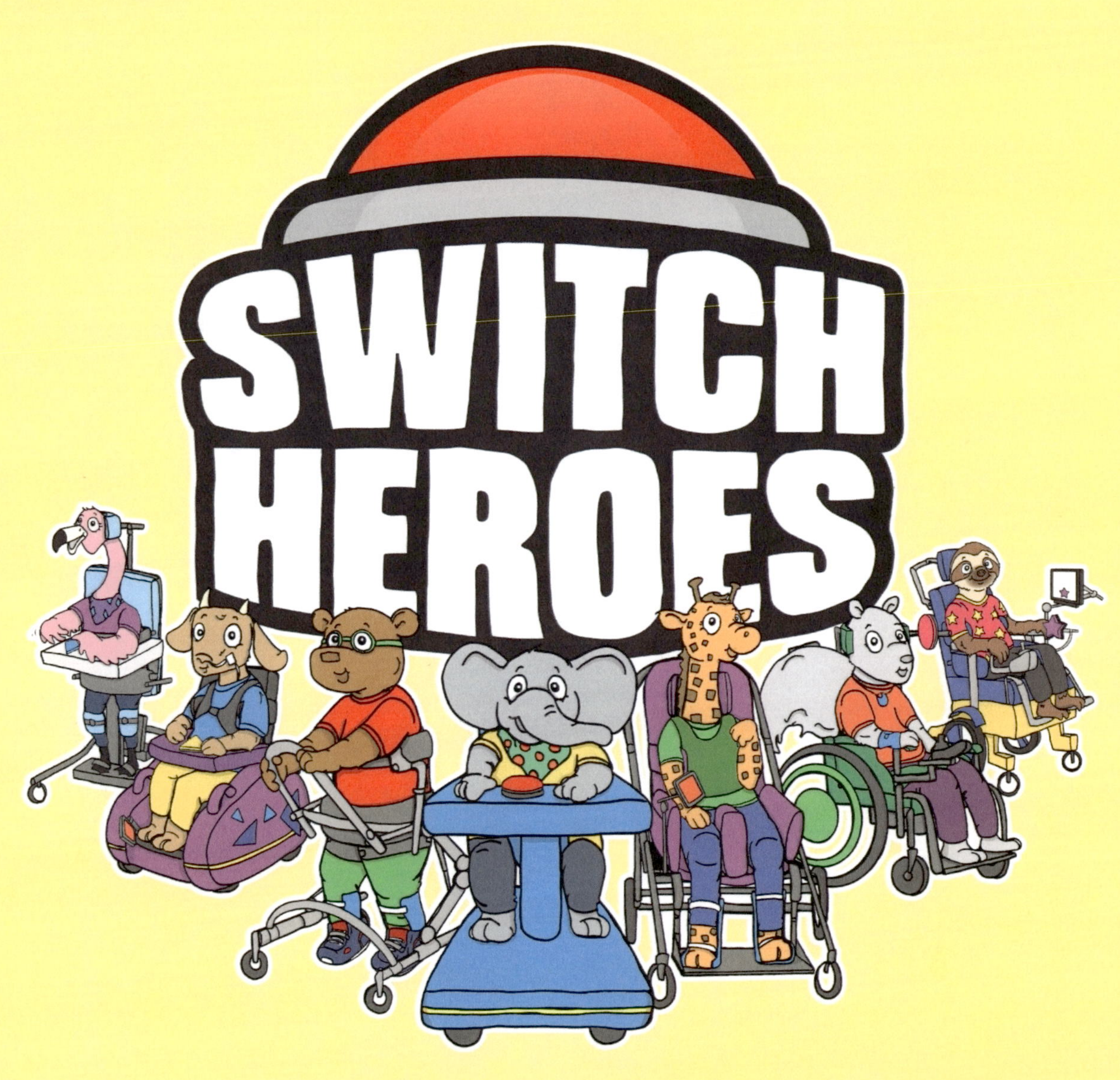
SWITCH
HEROES

The Seven Stages of Switch Development

The Seven Stages of Switch Development is a resource designed for switch-users, their families, caregivers and those who assist them in using switches. It features child-friendly characters and stories that support everyones learning.

The framework provides a helpful reference for measuring and tracking progress while offering flexibility to accommodate the unique needs and preferences of each switch-user.

Written directly to the switch-user, the framework can be read to them if they are unable to read it themselves. Our aim is to ensure that those supporting the child/switch-user can prioritise the child's needs and perspective in the process of developing their switch skills. We have seen the impact of involving the child in the learning process. Seeking their input and feedback regularly empowers them to take an active role in their development and combat learned helplessness.

Adapted from: Bean, I. (2011). Switch Progression Learning Journeys Road Map. Inclusive Technology. Burkhart, L. (2018). Stepping Stones to Switch Access. Perspectives of the ASHA Special Interest Groups, 3(12), pp.33-44. doi:https://doi/10.1044/persp3.sig12.33.

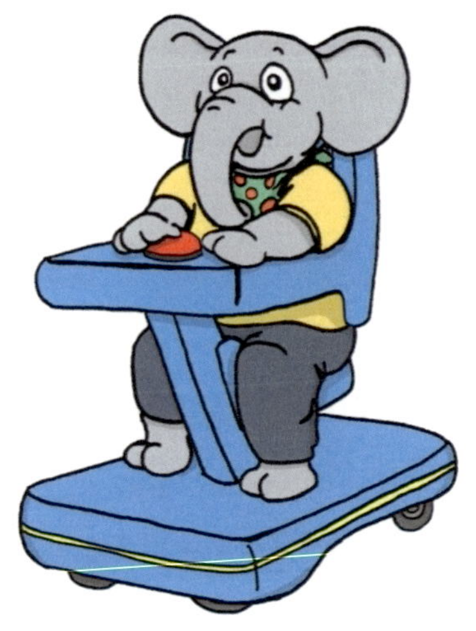

Definition

Exploring Egbert is the stage where you are first introduced to switches and learn how fun they can be. You will use your current easiest body movements, which could be your hand, arm, leg, head, or even your whole body moving forward. This will activate a switch that is placed where you can easily press it. Don't worry if it is not a smooth body movement, we will look at this at a later stage.

The switch location may be different depending on whether you are in a chair, lying down, standing in a standing frame, or a different position. The switch activation will give you either an instant or a very short timed sensory response (lights, sound, tactile, movement). It is important the activity is extremely fun and not complicated – no additional brain draining activities!

Through repeated opportunities to press your switch, you will learn, through experience that when you move your body and touch a switch (pressed or press and hold) a fun activity/response/reward happens.

Milestones

- Introduction to switches: you are introduced to switches and start to learn about their function and develop an acceptance to the equipment being near you

- Finding the easiest body movement: you can use your easiest body movement to activate the switch

- Incidental and curious switch activations: through repeated activations of the switch, you will learn that your body movements are causing a fun response

- Fun activities and rewards: as you continue to activate the switch you'll receive a fun activity or reward in response, such as lights, sound, tactile, or movement

- Provide frequent opportunities for the switch-user to use their switch across their day

- Ensure activities are fun, of interest and rewarding to the user

- Helpers can, if required, model what the switch does by pressing it to show the switch-user

- You can ask a therapist (e.g. Occupational Therapist or Physiotherapist) for advice on which body movement would be easiest for the switch-user to access their switch

- Try moving the switch closer to the switch-user or to somewhere they may incidentally activate it - avoid prompting at this stage as it shifts the child's focus from independent exploration to compliance

- Try different switches to see which one works best for the switch-user - do not get distracted by obsessing over getting the 'right' switch - there isn't one - just the best switch for the moment

- Consider the user's sensory needs when exploring the type of switch and switch activity (e.g. the clicking noise or the tactile feel of the switch can become a positive or negative focus)

- Communicate with the switch-user what happens when they use the switch with words, pictures or sounds

- Ensure activities involve direct activation, where the switch is on when activated and off when released, OR momentary activation, where the switch plays for a timed period (set for no longer than 6 seconds).

- Try using a switch that does something itself when it is pressed, such as light up or vibrate so the child can experience direct feedback

- Use cause and effect toys, for example, toys that activate a sound, light or movement when the switch is pressed. You could try a noisy switch toy to capture the child's attention

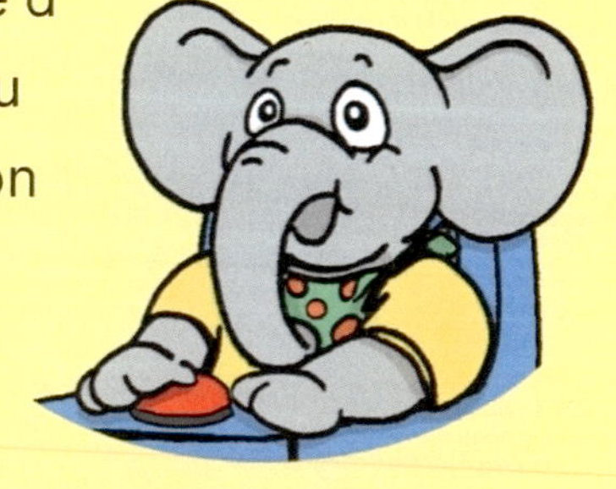

- Consider sensory activities, for example activities that provide sensory stimulation when the switch is pressed, such as bubble tubes, fibre optic lights, or vibrating toys

- Have a simple message recorded on a voice output switch that gives a simple, fun request, such as 'more tickles'. When the recording is played, ensure the response is given immediately

Instead of a prompt hierarchy where the type of prompt increase in support level, we recommend our one prompt switch support cycle. Find out more at Jiao.life

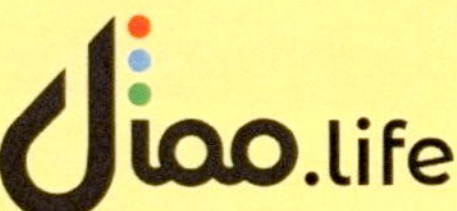

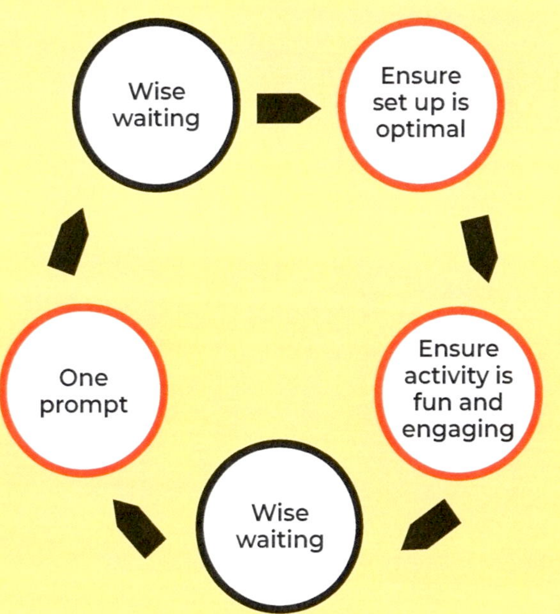

The Assessment Tool

Proficient step							
Consolidating step							
Emerging step							
Emerging – Developing – Consolidating – Proficient (cognitive, physical skill required for each stage)							
Physical	E D C P	E D C P	E D C P	E D C P	E D C P	E D C P	E D C P
Cognitive	E D C P	E D C P	E D C P	E D C P	E D C P	E D C P	E D C P

The Seven Stages of Switch Development ▶

Stage 1 Exploring Egbert	Stage 2 Journeying Jiao	Stage 3 Growing Gareth	Stage 4 Budding Brayton	Stage 5 Flourishing Fatima	Stage 6 Succeeding Saffi	Stage 7 Celebrating Syed
Learning by experience – single switch	Making something happen – single switch	Playing with two switches Making two things happen	Two switches one activity	Switch scanning – failure Free	Switch scanning – finding the right one	Independent in functional switch use

Print version available at 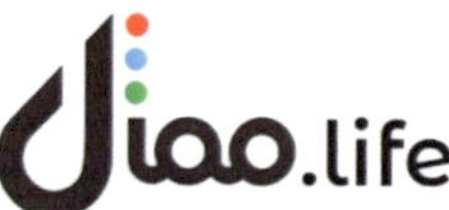

How to use the assessment tool

- The stages of switch development are not mutually exclusive, so progress can be made across multiple stages simultaneously

- Once a step is completed, mark it off and add the date

- The assessment tool can be used for goal setting, where helpers can add target dates and change the text/box colour accordingly

- There is a stream for assessing cognitive and physical skill development, divided into four steps for each stage (Emerging, Developing, Consolidating and Proficient)

- Helpers should consider the cognitive and physical skills required for each level

- This additional stream can help identify areas that may require additional support and highlight strengths and weaknesses for targeted interventions

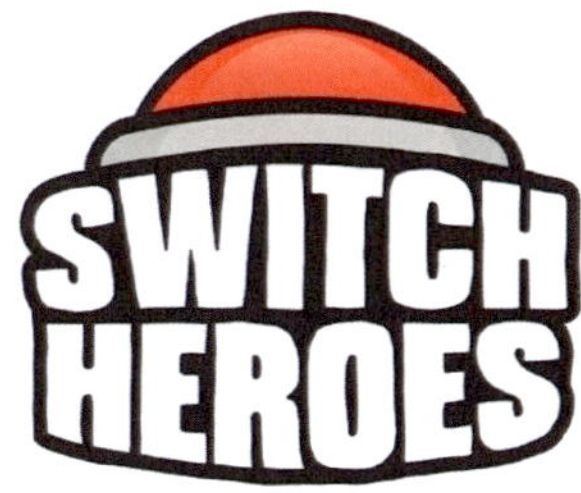

At Jiao Ltd, we are dedicated to empowering individuals through innovative assistive technology solutions.

We provide personalised services and training to help children, families, and professionals navigate the world of assistive tech. For more resources, training options, or to learn how we can support you, visit Jiao.life or get in touch with us directly. We look forward to hearing from you!

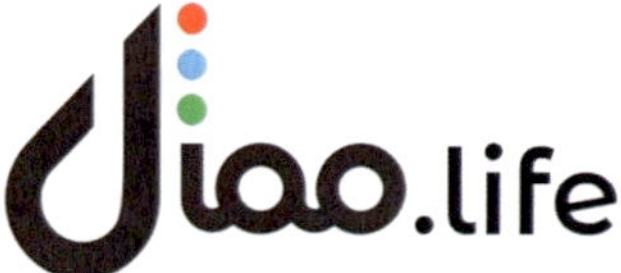

This is to certify that

____

is learning
by experience

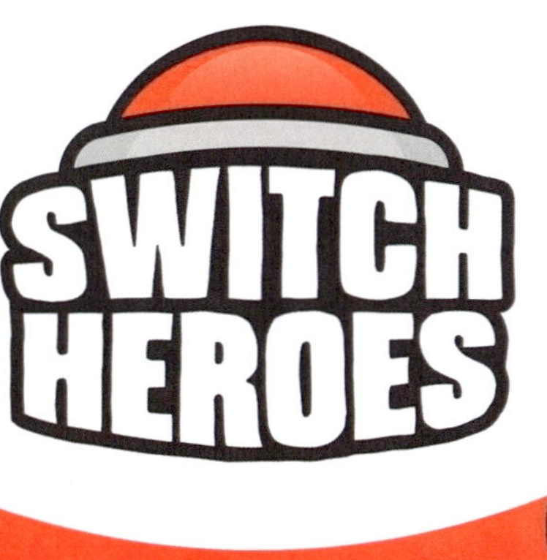

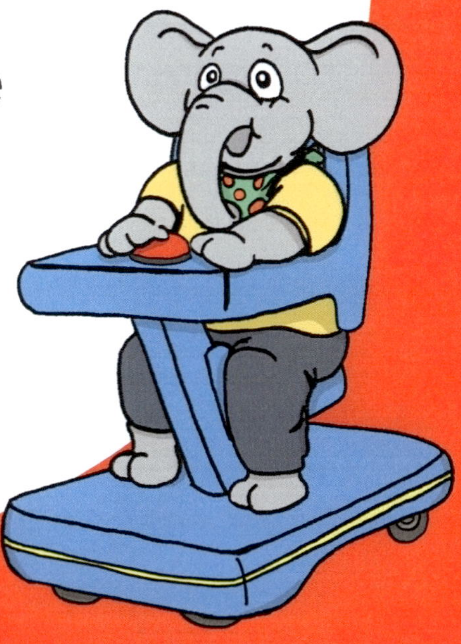

Notes